KEEP FIT

REGULAR EXERCISE BENEFITS TO LEAD A
HEALTHY LIFE

Exercise Definition

Regular exercise is one of the formulas for maintaining good health. Specifically, regular exercise can strengthen the heart, thereby reducing the risk of heart attack, stroke, high blood pressure, osteoporosis also obesity, it will also help in lessening the back pain. It also helps to combat unwanted stress and is a good way of relaxing or letting off steam; mitigating the risk of depression.

Studies show that performing half an hour at least three times a week in aerobic activity, and various muscle stretching and strengthening exercises at least two times a week to maximize your overall health benefits. Nevertheless, you can also achieve significant health benefits by performing a moderate-intensity physical activity for half an hour or more a day, at least five times a week.

If you just started in an exercise program, keep in mind to start at a slow pace with low-impact activities like walking, cycling, and swimming. These activities will improve your physical fitness level while safeguarding you from unwanted overuse burnout and injuries. You can progressively swap to varied and strenuous activities once your body adapts to it.

Does Regular Exercise Help in Health?

You may have heard of exercise quotes, to enjoy the glow of good health, you must exercise. However, how does exercise affect your overall health? Are the health benefits of exercise worth the effort it takes to exercise regularly? Can we choose to eat better instead of regular exercise to maintain our health? Is this a myth to have regular exercise to keep your health?

Here we give you reasons to consider taking exercise as part and parcel of your healthy lifestyle: According to a survey, Americans spend about 600 billion dollars on healthcare every year. This mentioned figure is equivalent to almost $3,000 for each of the whole population of the United States. Sadly, there is no sign of reduction in this financial commitment base on a yearly statistic. The factors which have been significant contributions to the widespread of medical problems in our society today are things like poor eating habits, lack of sleep, stress, abnormal lifestyle, poor health habits such as excessive smoking and drinking.

Meanwhile, studies have been conducted on the possibility to reduce either the number or mitigate the seriousness of the medical problems affecting society. These studies have concluded that exercise regularly has substantial medical benefits for people in different age groups. People who are physically active shows signs of improvement in longevity and reduced risk of heart disease. Low physical fitness and physical inactivity are the root cause of significant health problems. Exercise is medicine!

Let's agree with the mindset that regular exercise can play an essential role in lowering your risk of getting any medical problem, and avoiding your overall health care costs is one of the critical concerns. In general, exercise can partially treat and control most of the medical conditions and issues.

Below are some health concerns and recommended training to address and relieve each matter.

Allergies: Regular exercise can help to control allergies. The physical activity can improve the blood flow, and it will allow allergens to quickly move through the body and eliminated through the skin and kidneys.

Angina: Regular aerobic exercise can help to relieve chest pain as the workout can improve the blood flow. Consult a specialist or doctor on the type aerobic exercise that suits you the most and does it carefully to prevent any harm to your chest.

Anxiety: Exercise can produce chemicals like endorphins, and serotonin. Endorphins have the same effect to a painkiller to combat the depression, whereas serotonin will increase during and after an exercise. The increased levels of serotonin in the brain can fight anxiety and depression. This chemical can also help in sleep and improve self-esteem.

Arthritis: Exercise can increase flexibility and strength, and can help to relieve fatigue and reduce joint pain.

Back pain: Exercise can help to strengthen the stomach, back, and abdominal muscles — Regular training helps to support the spine and relieving back pain.

Cholesterol: Exercise will increase the levels of high-density lipoprotein (HDL is also known as good cholesterol) and also reduction in the levels of low-density lipoprotein (LDL is also known as bad cholesterol) in the blood.

Diabetes: Exercise can help in controlling the weight, improving the circulation and lowering excess blood sugar levels.

Heart disease: Exercise can help in lowering blood pressure and reducing strain on the heart, improving the heart, lung and liver efficiencies. Increasing the levels of HDL and reducing the levels of LDL result in mitigating the risk of heart problems.

Other diseases: Exercise can improve or heal both severe and minor illnesses. Regular exercise will reduce the risk of having cancers and stroke.

Knee problems: exercise can strengthen the muscles, ligaments, and tendons that support the joint. Stronger muscles can help the joint withstand the shock.

Menstrual problems and Premenstrual syndrome (PMS): Exercise can help in improving hormonal imbalances often associated with PMS. Exercise can relieve menstrual pain, bloating and cramping.

Osteoporosis: Exercise can strengthen muscles and build bone, increase bone density to mitigate the risk of bone fracture.

Overweight problems: Exercise can increase lean muscle mass and metabolic rate. It can also burn fat. Many scientific types of research prove that regular exercise can contribute to weight loss especially the number of burnt calories more than consumed from nutrition. You can get rid of the unwanted fat if you exercise regularly and control diet.

Social capabilities: Exercise can boost self-esteem, and help you look better and more active in meeting people. It will prevent you from feeling unsupported and isolated. Exercising will also promote the interests in sex in improving your marriage relationship.

Wellness and mentality: Exercise can build up your confidence when you are in great shape. You will be motivated and energetic which can help you to be more productive in everything. Exercising can help create a sense of direction to improve your focus to accomplish the goals that you might think is impossible. Regular exercise can also help you to increase the levels of perseverance; it will prevent you from going off track while moving towards your goal.

How to Enjoy Exercise

There are three main basics that are essential to make any exercise program work. They are safety, effectiveness, and enjoyment.

Safety: The "No pain, no gain" theory does not fully apply to this topic. Keep in mind to avoid any exercise that will cause injury, undue discomfort or pain. Cease all exercises and to seek immediate medical attention if there is any pain occurs in any part of your body.

General muscle aching is familiar especially for the beginner. You probably will experience some bearable aching when you get started to workout. A personal trainer will plan an exercise program for you based on your present fitness levels. Your fitness programme will be adjusted according to your fitness progress in due course, so you are to do it step by step. Excessive exercise will eventually undermine your efforts.

Using the proper form and right technique to avoid any high-impact to keep your exercise program safe. A sprain in your back or joints is an inevitable result of improper form or technique. Jarring and repetitive movements should avoid for general fitness.

Do not force or bounce stretching movements. Pulsing and quick changes while stretching are likely to cause muscle tears or strains. For general fitness stretching, it is recommended to do static stretching that gradually extend your muscles until you feel resistance. Stretching is suppleness of joints and muscles to enable the increased effectiveness during exercise, and it will also decrease the likelihood of injury and arching.

Effectiveness: Effective exercise requires effort; your level of fitness and goals determine the level of physical activity. Persevere to the recommended exercises and level of intensity to achieve the expected result if you are aiming to get rid of the excess body fat. Weight, Intensity, repetitions and rest periods should adjust according to your fitness progress. Proper stretching and warm up before exercising and cool down afterward is vital to avoid any internal or external injury and achieve peak performance.

Enjoyment: Apart from knowing that we can gain from exercise, we also need additional motivation or goals for us to achieve the best result from regular exercise.

It is essential to determine your direction and goal that you want to achieve so your exercising effort can be focused on your goal(s) to keep it motivated. The more motivated you are, the more enjoyable it is. Motivation can be exchangeable with enjoyment especially you can see the significant result either in stamina or better shape. Treating exercise like playing a game or activities you used to enjoy during early childhood. If possible, to find a partner who can exercise with you to have some interaction.

Making Exercise More Fun

A minority is willing to reduce their bedtime in the morning with the thought of going for exercise. After a hectic day, you probably will not think of doing some workout in a gym room or a simple jog. Sometimes, you might think of exercising at home, but the fitness equipment is limited.

Occasionally, you cannot overcome the state of sluggishness, inactivity, and apathy to get motivated to exercise on a regular basis. You may find exercise can be bored and downright dull at times. You may be pondering how to be motivated to keep yourself persevere in exercising on a regular basis. You can discover several fun ideas that can be integrated into your exercise to make it more enjoyable.

1) You should exercise with friends. You can compete with each other, help each other to achieve the fitness goal, mutually encouragement and make each other laugh or create some games out of your exercise programs.

2) You can also try something different; try mixing things up. For example, using the same piece of equipment in the gym room and the same part of the equipment at home.

3) Changing the order of your exercises or reverse your routine may be deemed necessary.

4) You can go to a park that provides playground equipment and use the slide, hang from your knees, do pull-ups and climb on the monkey bars, and do it freely. You do not always need to stick to a routine, get out there and get some fun in the exercise.

5) You also can try some outdoor circuits in the park. Some parks provide the circuit courses set up with a planned route; you can follow the instruction provided by either walking or jogging to each station. If the park does not give any scheduled course, you consider doing a combination of walking and jogging, picking a distance of multiple of a hundred feet. Walk 100 feet then drop and do 20 push-ups, jog the next 100 feet and then drop to do 20 sit-ups.

6) You can cycle around your area or hike on a hiking trail. A jog around your neighborhood or in the park is also a great way to get some exercise. Doing yoga on a beach or in the park is also another relaxing and pleasant option to exercise your body and mind.

7) You also can think of participating in a competitive sport. Many cities will have team activities such as basketball, volleyball, badminton, tennis, soccer, etc. These types of games will provide you with good exercise also help you to know friends as well.

8) Always try to visualize your muscles are developing and getting more prominent when you exercise. Research has shown that the muscles will form better if you keep focusing all of your attention on them that you are working. Try to monitor the muscles with each repetition as they contract and relax.

As you notice there are many ways you can make exercise more fun and exciting. You do not need to stick to the same routine day after day, as you can be involved in other activities to get into exercise. The important thing is you should always try to integrate exercise in any various form into your daily life and habituate yourself to exercise.

Exercise as Power Source

Your busy schedule might create a challenge to persevere in exercise each day. Our exercise objective is releasing stress and boosting the body with extra energy so we can carry out a healthy lifestyle. You can see the significant and noticeable results of exercise with perseverance coupled with refined techniques, cardio, functional activities, variety, awareness, the right nutrition and motivation over some time.

The refined techniques mean a correct form to isolate muscles or to target areas of the body. Efficiency needs to ensure the contract and relax (stimulation) of the muscles. You will need to get rid of any momentum in weight lift training known as resistance training. It is also important to lift the weight by using a full range of motion. Full range of motion helps to ensure the correct length of the tendons and cause the muscle to contract for the suitable timing. The activity is to strengthen the joints of your body and muscles.

Cadence, also known as tempo, is also helpful as it is a term that refers to the rate in which the weight moves or resistance. You can achieve the best results with cadence by doing in slow movements which will make the muscle in a contract mode for a longer time. You can do a mixture of fast and slow cadence, which is very useful in the training. Adopting the correct angles will achieve muscle isolation in target areas and help to reduce the risk of injuries, which is good for those using heavyweights.

Functional type exercise is a favorite way that will stimulate the torso and core of your body while you are working on another muscle group simultaneously. For example, to lift the dumbbell while lying on an exercise ball. Your core muscles and the abdominal muscles will contract to hold your body into this position, while your chest and triceps muscles will lift the dumbbells. This type of workout will cause supreme stimulation to your body and keep the exercise refreshing and motivating.

Cardio is an alternative exercise that is good for the heart and lungs. The total calories burnt is significant along with maintaining the right heart rate. Below are the rules of thumb to keep track your healthy heart rate.

Lower figure: 220 minus your age times 60
Upper figure: 220 minus your age times 80

Cardio is also known as the fat burning zone. Cardio will help to boost the immune system and make you feel better; it will also detoxify the body. The muscles will contract and relax, and pass the lymph along, which will improve and allow the immune system to replace the dead cells.

Warming up is very important before exercise. Performing a warm-up will prepare your body for any demanding workout of cardio. You should always do at least 15 minutes warm-up before weightlifting, and a minimum of 10 minutes before cardio exercises.

Stretching is equally important as a warm-up, performing the muscle stretching will help in blood circulation and allow the blood flowing through the muscles. Doing warm-up and stretching is a must before cardio. To achieve a better result, you can lift weights in every other day starting from Monday followed by Wednesday, and then Friday, then do cardio only on Tuesday and Thursday.

Even though you may think your day is too hectic to maintain a plan for any physical training, you will find that adding exercise will eat into your time and physical activity will consume lots of your energy. You can imagine physical activity is acting like the batteries to replenish the lost power.

Exercise at Home with Videos

Nowadays, there are a lot of people buying exercise videos. There are a variety of exercise videos in the market. Are there any advantages in using exercise videos? Well, in a word, yes, there are a lot of benefits by watching exercise videos to guide you.

There are exercise videos made for home workouts. Home workouts offer a lot of benefits over going to the gym. For instance, you can choose to exercise at home at your timing, and you do not have to worry that the gym is crowded or is the fitness equipment occupied by others. You do not need to worry about punctuality attending the scheduled fitness class. You can choose any exercise attire that you want, and you will feel comfortable while exercising at all times. A point to note is always to select the proper sports attire and gear that protects you. Furthermore, there are many free videos can be found from online, you can bookmark and subscribe to the particular channel if you deem the videos helpful. And also save time by skipping the unnecessary time driving to the gym room.

Exercise videos come with a variety of workouts including burn fat, build muscle, release stress, circuit workouts, flexibility (stretching and yoga), balance exercises (Tai Chi), and even mental exercise like meditation — a variety of different styles like dancing, kickboxing, step aerobics, Pilates, jump rope, and many more to name that are available in exercise videos.

The exercise videos are available from amateur to expert level in the market. It is vital for you to select the ones that suit you the most. You can even find the videos for specific purposes such as workouts for seniors, adult, children, pregnant women and those suffering from back pain. You can select those exercise videos that do not require any fitness equipment or choose the ones that use the necessary fitness items such as a dumbbell, mini-trampolines, rubber tubing, aerobic steps, stability balls, and body bars and or the home gym multi-stations. It is not hard to find a video that demonstrates relating to the equipment that you have. The fitness equipment can be easily found any major department stores and sports stores.

Exercise videos are your perfect tools in guiding you throughout your home workouts in variable intensity levels and types of exercise that your body can take it. It is paramount to conform strictly to the played exercise video and exercising while watching the video. You will not achieve any results if you are merely sitting on the sofa watching the exercise video. Perseverance is vital to making a noticeable effect.

You can Exercise in the Office

We spent most of our time sitting down. Sitting at home for breakfast, when you commute to work, the whole day in the office, traveling back home and sitting down again at home in the evening again. More often than not, sitting in the office takes up more than 50 percent of the time spent on sitting.

Moreover, in modern lifestyle, there's never seemed to have sufficient time for you to do all the things that you need to do and yet find time to workout. However, spending long hours in front of your computer doesn't mean that it is impossible to find time to exercise and keep fit. These 6-office workouts will enable you to stay fit even when you are stuck in your office:

1. **Chair Crunches**

- Sit near to the end of the chair and lie back to the backrest.
- Both arms are gripping firmly at the side of the chair.

- Lift your feet off the floor and move your knees up toward your chest.
- Straighten your legs out without touching the floor

This is considered as one rep. Complete 10 reps for beginners, 20 reps for intermediate, and 30 reps for advanced.

2. Seated Triceps Liftbacks

- Sit upright with your back firmly on the chair backrest.
- Hold a 1.5 liters bottle with both hands and lift it above your head. Keep your arms straight.
- Lower the bottle until your arms are at 90 degrees angle.
- Straighten your arms again.

This is considered as one rep. Complete 10 reps for beginners, 20 reps for intermediate, and 30 reps for advanced.

3. Squat Calf Raise

- Stand at the back of your chair and both hands holding on the chair as support.
- Bent your knees to an angle of 90 degrees.
- Maintaining this posture, stand on your tiptoes and hold it for three seconds.

- Return to the bent knee position.

This is considered as one rep. Complete 10 reps for beginners, 20 reps for intermediate, and 30 reps for advanced.

4. Chair Plank

- Place both your forearms onto the seat of the chair.
- Extend your body until it forms a straight line and contracts your abdominal muscles.
- Hold this position for 30 seconds.
- Ensure that your body maintains a straight line throughout the workout.

Complete one rep for beginners, two reps for intermediate, and three reps for advanced.

5. Desk Pushups

- Place both your hands on your table.
- Without removing your hands from the table, more approximately 5 feet away from your desk.
- Lower yourself until your chest is almost touching your table and hold the position for one second.
- Straighten both arms.

This is considered as one rep. Complete 10 reps for beginners, 20 reps for intermediate, and 30 reps for advanced.

6. Squats

- Stand in front of your table, and both hands are holding onto the table as support.
- Squat down until your leg is at an angle of around 30 degrees.
- Stand back up until the starting position.

This is considered as one rep. Complete 10 reps for beginners, 20 reps for intermediate, and 30 reps for advanced.

These six workouts will count as one set. Complete 1 set for beginners, two sets for intermediate, and three sets for advanced.

With this quick and simple, yet effective office workout, you can maintain a toned body and at the same time complete all your work within the given deadline. **You can make use of a quarter of your lunchtime or tea break to do this workout in the office, and also helpful to your back especially we are sitting for the whole day during office hour.** One thing to note is that such exercise is not advisable right after your meals.

It is also vital that you have the right posture while sitting. You back must be straight, shoulders to the back, knees should be at an angle of 90 degrees, feet flat on the ground, maintain a reasonable distance between you and your computer screen, and head should be upright while you are using the computer. You will reduce the risk of getting back and neck pain, thus improving productivity.

Additional Benefits from Exercise:

Exercise can help with anti-aging. Many people are willing to invest in a new form of treatment which is anti-aging. There are a few popular treatments such as injectables; the injected chemical can give useful and instant results in reducing wrinkles and fine lines of the face. Another popular treatment for our skin, also known as chemical peel treatment, is done by applying a type of chemical directly to the skin surface, and it will cause the skin to burn and eventually become the dead skin cells to peel off. Lastly will be a popular laser treatment; it improves the overall wellness of the skin, targeting fine lines, scars, skin tone, and texture. The laser damages the skin and lets the skin reborn with the help in collagen promotion. Your skin is likely experiencing agitated, swelling or feeling pain after the anti-aging treatments.

Today, we will focus on the injectable of the Anti-Aging Treatments. Skin specialist or doctor will inject the Human Growth Hormone (which known as HGH) and doses of nutrient supplements to your skin. There are alternative natural ways to improve your skin from exercising and dieting. Studies have shown that strength training will help to promote and produce HGH. Strength training is specifically stimulating to specific muscle growth. You can do simple weight lifting by using dumbbells either in the gym room or home, or do some squatting will strengthen your bottom part of your body muscles to produce HGH. At the same time, you can lose weight by doing a workout. Workout merely takes you about half an hour a day and three times a week.

Studies also discovered that your body would produce $10,000 worth of beneficial chemicals that the body needs for every hour throughout the workout. You may not require to undergo any anti-aging treatments if you exercise regularly as your body will produce the useful chemical naturally.

Try to be self-discipline to adhere to regular exercise and strength training. Apart from gaining the HGH, the training will improve in your bone mass, and allow more oxygen to your body tissues and organ for well-functioning. You will also feel energetic after a few months of regular exercise as you can control your weight and bring more oxygen to your both brain and body. Instead of going for HGH injections that make more HGH, physical activities can achieve the same or better results in a more natural way. Hence, give it a try to produce the HGH that your body needs by doing physical activities regularly.

Exercise regularly will bring you the best result in rejuvenating the skin and a great looking body. It will be great if the training can couple with a healthy diet, it will also possibly prolong your life.

For diet wise, always go for the healthier choice, and to consume everything in moderation. Try to cut down eating red meats, refined sugar, salt, and fats but to have more fruits especially berries, whole grains, fishes but not shellfish to complete your meal menu. You will gradually be energetic and feeling better after you change your diet habit. The new diet habit coupled with exercises will help to control weight.

Also, you can have additional natural nutritional supplements to ensure the needed essential nutrients are adequate. The natural dietary supplements will help in the anti-aging process.

Exercise can Improve your Complexion

As we know that exercise can make you lose weight, firm your muscles, build stamina, and contribute in energy, making you stay healthy. You might not know that exercise can also improve your complexion.

Studies have proven that regular exercise will rejuvenate your skin with the help of new blood, oxygen and essential nutrients in the body. It will increase blood flow and improve blood circulation to detoxify your body to strengthen the vital organs and epidermis.

There are a lot of misconceptions that sweat is harmful to our skin and will form the acne flare-ups. It is not true. Sweating is suitable for any skin type as it will help promote the flushing of impurities from the surface to rinse your skin. Vigorous exercise will also improve your hormonal imbalances that can cause hair loss, weight gain, and fatigue. Jogging, hiking, cycling, and yoga or any physical activities that you like will help to reduce the stress that you face every day to prevent stress-related acne outbreak. However, do note that exercise may is not a cure for all your skin problems. You may still experience breakouts occasionally. However, the acne will be less severe as compared to without any exercising.

Exercise is also benefiting other skin conditions apart from the acne problem. It will also firm your skin. Our skin will lose the elasticity and become less resilient when we get old; this is a common issue for the elderly. Collagen is slowly losing when our age diminishes. Many of us may not know that physical activities can help to promote the growth of collagen in the skin cells, which can regain the skin radiant and make you look younger.

You can even have a smaller waist, better build, smoother skin, and a younger and fresher look. Hence hesitate no more if you wish to improve your complexion. Just cater an hour for the workout for you to be more energetic and livelier.

Exercise to Make You Sleep Better

Some people may have a hard time sleeping during the night or taking a nap during the daytime. These people will either find it hard to sleep on the bed, keep waking up after a while or is a light sleeper. As a result, they will feel either exhausted and fatigue after waking up.

Exercise can improve the quality of sleep, the amount of physical activity that you do in the daytime is one of the critical factors to help you sleep well at night. The more energy that you use up during the workout, the more likely you can be asleep faster and sleep well at night. You will discover that your quality of sleep will be better and the transition between the phases and cycles of rest will be regular and smoother with the help of regular exercise.

Studies have found out that there is a direct correlation between the amount of energy that used in the workout and how we feel after exercise. You will feel that you have more energy when you exercise more often. One of the key reasons is because exercise can combat stress and worries of your life. Hence, you should start planning the exercise program and try to allow more time for you to exercise in the daytime. The reason to do that is to give your body enough stimulation in the daytime, so you are not full of energy during night time. You require a certain amount of exercise to keep the vital organs functioned healthily. It is recommended to avoid any physical activities 4 hours before you go to bed.

The best exercise time is before evening time. You need to make sure the energy that you use in the physical activity is long enough before you rest or sleep. You should plan to exercise at least every other day for a minimum of 30 minutes. You can consider some simple workout like walking or jogging. The objective to do that is to strengthen your vital organs like heart and lungs. It will also improve the heart rate, the capacity of the lungs and overall health and help in emotion by adding in the regular physical activity to your daily schedule.

Apart from walking and jogging, there are many other physical activities that you can consider adding into your regular activity schedule. You can think of doing the aerobic exercise if you do not have any problem in your sleep. Aerobic exercise refers to any physical activities that require oxygen, and it will increase your heart and breathing rate during the aerobic activities. You can choose any one of the aerobic exercises that you like the most and suit you the most. The events include jogging, running, cycling, dancing, jumping rope, etc.

Of course, there are other non-aerobic exercises that you may find it beneficial to address your sleeping problem, and we merely focus on Yoga and Ta Chi in this book.

1. Yoga

Yoga is an exercise that can benefit both your mind and body. Let's start with the mind; yoga has a stimulatory effect on the nervous system especially the brain's nervous system. Yoga uses the breathing techniques and yoga postures to increase and improve the blood circulation to the body and mind, promoting regular, relaxing and restful sleeping patterns. The daily yoga will help you to stay calm and relax as well as relieve worry and stress. Yoga also helps you to manage stress, which is known to have devastating effects on both mind and body.

Next is to talk about the physical benefits of practicing yoga. Maintaining a regular yoga practice with relaxation techniques can relieve chronic pain like back pain, arthritis carpal tunnel syndrome, and headaches, and also increase flexibility, muscle strength, and tone, and improve respiration, vitality, and energy. One of the great benefits from yoga is to lower blood pressure.

2. Tai Chi

Tai Chi is a non-competitive martial art known for its self-defense techniques. It is also an ancient art of breathing and movement that was developed by Chinese monks. Tai Chi's actions are slow and precise, it combines gentle physical exercise and stretching with mindfulness.

Tai Chi is the perfect exercise for people who have joint pains or unable to participate in high aerobic physical activities especially elderly as the Tai Chi action is safe for all ages, as it does stress the muscles and joints.

Tai Chi can also improve balance, relieve pain and the symptoms of depression in some cases, enhanced the immune system and promote relaxation helping with insomnia.

Conclusion

Thank you for your precious time to read this book. You should make the best effort to exercise and make it a part of your lifestyle. You can achieve good results from the regular exercise, and your healthy lifestyles depend on how intensive the training is.

After knowing all of the benefits and reasons to exercise, you should not have any hesitation about exercise. You can decide either exercise at home with the guidance of an exercise video or go to the gym room under the supervision of a personal trainer.

There are many ways that we can exercise, merely choosing the physical activities that you like the most. Slowly increase the time and fitness levels when your body starts to adapt to the routine. You will feel much better and your body will eventually thank you. So, wait no more, please plan your exercise program now!

If you enjoyed this book and found some benefit in reading this, I'd like to hear from you and hope that you could take some time to post a review on Amazon. Your feedback and support will help this author to greatly improve his writing craft for future projects and make this book even better

You can follow this link to **[Book link here]** now.

I want you, the reader, to know that your review is very important and so, if you'd like to **leave a review**, all you have to do is click **[Link here]** and away you go. I wish you all the best in your future success!

www.ingramcontent.com/pod-product-compliance
Lightning Source LLC
Chambersburg PA
CBHW051136250726
48655CB00007B/3098